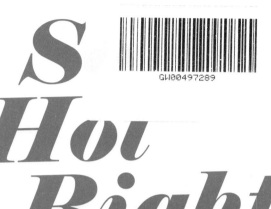

# So Hot Right Now

SO HOT RIGHT NOW

Text by Sam Lacey

An Hachette UK Company
www.hachette.co.uk

Vie Books, an imprint of Summersdale Publishers Ltd
Part of Octopus Publishing Group Limited
Carmelite House
50 Victoria Embankment
LONDON
EC4Y 0DZ
UK

www.summersdale.com

Printed and bound in China

ISBN: 978-1-80007-709-6

Substantial discounts on bulk quantities of Summersdale books are available to corporations, professional associations and other organizations. For details contact general enquiries: telephone: +44 (0) 1243 771107 or email: enquiries@summersdale.com.

# So Hot Right Now

Peer-reviewed by Dr Samantha Sanders, health psychologist

## The Little Book of Perimenopause

**ALEX GREENGATE**

# Disclaimer

The author and the publisher cannot accept responsibility for any misuse or misunderstanding of any information contained herein, or any loss, damage or injury, be it health, financial or otherwise, suffered by any individual or group acting upon or relying on information contained herein. None of the views or suggestions in this book is intended to replace medical opinion from a doctor who is familiar with your particular circumstances. If you have concerns about your health, please seek professional advice.

# Contents

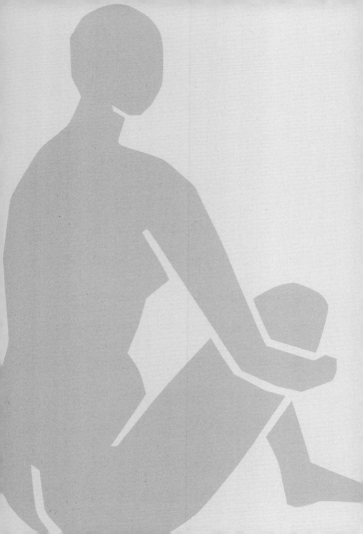

# Introduction

The chances are that if you've picked up this book, you may have looked at the title and thought, "Well, that's me – and not in a good way!" Is that right? You might be experiencing the best known symptom, hot flushes, as well as other changes to your body, mood, sleep pattern, libido, anxiety levels... the list goes on. But fear not! All kinds of unusual things can start happening as we approach menopause. And the lead up to the menopause itself (known as the perimenopause) can begin at a much earlier age than we might think or expect – anywhere from the mid-thirties to the early fifties, while the average age is 45–47. However, none of the changes you might be going through, or may experience in the future, are anything to worry about. Some of us will sail through this phase in our life, and others may not. Whichever camp you fall into, and however you experience any changes, this book is here to help. It's filled to the brim with information about what's going on and lots of advice on how to deal with it. So grab your favourite brew (and perhaps a chocolate biscuit) and settle down to find out more.

# Perimenopause and menopause should be treated as the rites of passage that they are.

GILLIAN ANDERSON

# Chapter One

## *Understanding Perimenopause*

So, what exactly *is* perimenopause? You may never have even heard of this term, and now you might be wondering whether you are in it! Everyone will have a different experience, so this chapter will take a deeper look at what perimenopause is, how it may affect you, how you might recognize the symptoms and when you might expect it – as well as some common myths and misconceptions. Also, rather helpfully, it will explain how you can prepare for its arrival.

# Perimenopause: an overview

Most of us have probably heard of the menopause. More than likely, we expect to go through it when we are "older" – at least during our fifties. At times you might have experienced symptoms that could be menopausal, but thought: this *surely* can't be the menopause? I'm far too young! Well, yes *and* no. You are considered to have gone through the menopause itself when you have not had a menstrual period for 12 months, meaning that your ovaries no longer produce any eggs. However, many changes in our bodies can begin to happen gradually over time before we arrive at the menopause. These changes often start from a reasonably young age – typically in our forties, but sometimes even earlier, in our thirties. This time leading up to menopause is known as the perimenopause (meaning "around the menopause") and is essentially the journey to menopause. Postmenopause ("after the menopause") lasts for the rest of your life, and some perimenopause symptoms can linger for several years after periods have stopped.

Perimenopause is kicked off when levels of oestrogen and progesterone, the two key female hormones, begin to drop. As well as hot flushes (or flashes), tiredness, forgetfulness and a range of other physical and psychological changes (more on those later), one of the very first physical symptoms of perimenopause that you may notice is irregular periods. Your usual menstrual cycle can change, and periods might start to become a little erratic. Bleeding may get lighter or heavier, and the gaps between periods may become longer or shorter. This is all completely normal.

*Other conditions can cause irregular bleeding, so if you are at all concerned, do see a health practitioner to rule these out.*

# How do I tell if I am in perimenopause?

If you are experiencing unusual symptoms such as hot flushes, irregular periods, vaginal dryness, difficulty concentrating or feeling more tired than usual, you may well have entered perimenopause. If you would like confirmation of this, you can ask a medical professional to carry out a blood test to determine your levels of FSH (follicle-stimulating hormone). FSH is made in the pituitary gland and is higher during this time.

Once you've established that you are in it, you might wonder how long perimenopause will last. Your experience, and its duration, will be personal to you and you alone. However, to give an idea, perimenopause can last anywhere from a few months to several years. Although some days it might not feel like it, menopause and the years leading up to it are actually a cause for celebration; you are on the cusp of a new phase of your life.

# Preparing for change

Be grateful for your amazing body doing its thing and know that, while it will go through a bit of a change, you can help yourself by laying the groundwork to deal with it well. One of the best things you can do – at any age – is to keep healthy and look after your overall well-being. Exercise regularly, eat well, find time to relax, get enough sleep, invest in positive, nurturing relationships: all of this will help you to cope with any symptoms much better when they do arrive. The other thing that will help immensely, if you feel able to, is to talk about it. While your symptoms are individual to you, you may have friends going through perimenopause, too, so you might be able to share tips and give each other advice. Together you can help each other to get through this time and come out the other side sparkling, with a new and slightly different vitality.

# A quick look at hormones

As well as the two key female hormones of oestrogen and progesterone, our bodies also contain testosterone. All of these go into decline in the perimenopausal years. Before we look at some of the effects of lower levels of these hormones, here's a summary of what they do.

## *Oestrogen*

Most oestrogen is made in the ovaries, with a small amount also manufactured in the adrenal glands (which sit at the top of the kidneys) and in fat cells. Receptors are found throughout the whole body. Oestrogen's main job is to regulate periods, though it also affects the urinary tract, heart, blood vessels, brain, bones, breasts, skin, hair and pelvic muscles. It keeps cholesterol in check and is also linked to mood, as it increases serotonin receptors. It's no wonder, then, that when levels start to wane, we notice! If you cast your mind back to puberty, when oestrogen levels began to rise, this is what fuelled physical changes such as breast development, a widening waistline and the growth of body hair. Its decline, then, goes some way to explain why our hair can become thinner in the run-up to menopause.

## Progesterone

Also produced in the ovaries, another key hormone in our bodies is progesterone. It is often used in combination with oestrogen to treat perimenopause and menopause symptoms (see Chapter Three). Progesterone's main role in the body is to thicken mucus in the cervix, helping the body to prepare for pregnancy (if required). As levels drop, it can cause vaginal dryness, which in turn can mean that having sex is uncomfortable. We'll take a look at how to deal with this unwelcome side effect later in the book.

## Testosterone

This predominantly male hormone has a key role for everyone. Like oestrogen, it is produced in the ovaries and adrenal glands and affects libido, bone strength, mood and brain function. Although testosterone levels don't drop as suddenly as oestrogen and progesterone as we enter perimenopause, in females it reduces by half between the ages of 20 and 40 and continues to decline as we get older.

# Where are my glasses?!

It isn't just physical symptoms that can come about during perimenopause: replace "glasses" with anything: phone, keys, shoes, bag, doughnut... you get the idea. Fluctuations in hormone levels can make us absent-minded and cause brain fog – meaning we can find it difficult to concentrate. Researchers think this is because oestrogen helps with the growth of neurons, which send electrical impulses to our brain. Rest assured, though; studies have found that memory can return to more normal levels postmenopause. In the meantime, try to get into a routine of putting things in the same place: keys on the table, glasses and phone on the nightstand, shoes in the cupboard – and doughnuts, of course, belong in our stomach.

# Anxiety

Another psychological effect of perimenopause can be becoming worried or anxious – often about things that you normally wouldn't have given a second thought to. A trip to a new city for a team-building event might once have been something to be excited about, but as it rolls around, you just cannot face the journey or having to negotiate your way around; nor do you have the energy to meet new people. So you feign illness and don't go. There are some tips on how to manage anxiety in Chapter Two, and some treatments you could try in Chapter Three – but please don't worry if this is the new you. As with many things about perimenopause, it is temporary and doesn't affect everyone. Your social skills and *joie de vivre* will reappear in abundance!

*If you are concerned about anxiety, please don't suffer in silence. Pay a visit to your health professional for advice.*

# The heat is on!

Night sweats are a common occurrence in the perimenopausal years, though they are not restricted to night-time. They give a sudden feeling of heat in your body, sometimes travelling upward into your face, causing redness and sweating. They often depart as quickly as they arrive but can leave you feeling flustered. At night, they might wake you up and make it difficult to get back to sleep. Some things, such as caffeine and alcohol, can make hot flushes worse, so it might be worth keeping a note of what you've eaten or drunk to see if there's a pattern. And perhaps avoid that double-shot latte!

*Hot flushes are believed to be caused by changes in your brain's hypothalamus – your thermostat control – due to decreasing oestrogen. Thinking your body's too warm, the hypothalamus triggers blood vessels near the skin's surface to dilate, making you sweat. A "chill pillow" filled with cooling gel might give relief, or try slow abdominal breathing to help you through a hot flush.*

I've discovered that this is your moment to reinvent yourself after years of focusing on the needs of everyone else.

**OPRAH WINFREY**

# *Stimulate my follicles!*

Our hormones have a lot to answer for as they start to desert us, not least of which is changing the appearance and texture of our hair. If you start to find yours is becoming thinner and more difficult to manage, something as simple as changing to a thickening shampoo or a rich conditioner for dry hair may do the trick. Or you could try letting it dry naturally, as this is kinder than daily blow-drying and straightening; what your hair was prepared to tolerate when you were a little younger may be something it is no longer willing to accept. If your locks have lost their lustre, try a hair oil to restore sheen; if you find your hair is becoming really problematic, ask your hairstylist or a pharmacist for advice; or if you prefer to keep it natural, some studies suggest that a couple of drops of rosemary essential oil mixed into your shampoo may help protect against nerve damage and hair loss. It could even be that having your stylist give your hair a colour treatment might improve its condition and add some shine, as well as give you renewed confidence and sparkle.

# *Be still, my beating heart*

Have you noticed your heart sometimes beating a little faster? Even when you're *not* watching a shirtless Chris Hemsworth on Netflix? This could be another indicator of perimenopause. Variations in oestrogen levels can cause palpitations, which can occur either on their own or during a hot flush. They are usually pretty harmless, but if you are worried, talk to a health practitioner. Heart health in general is something to be aware of during perimenopause, as two of the roles of oestrogen in the body are controlling the build-up of plaque in your arteries and keeping cholesterol in check. Lower levels, therefore, can increase the risk of cardiovascular disease. Reducing alcohol intake, stopping smoking, taking regular exercise, managing stress levels and healthy eating are the best ways to protect your cardiovascular system; some treatments, including Hormone Replacement Therapy (HRT), are said to offer some protection against heart disease – more on this in Chapter Three.

# Women of colour

Although everyone's experience will be unique to them, one study has shown that women of colour tend to enter perimenopause earlier, have it last longer and are more likely to get night sweats and hot flushes. Black women in particular are three times more likely to start seeing symptoms before the age of 40, while Hispanic women often report an increased heart rate. As going through an earlier menopause has been linked to a possible longer-term risk to heart health, in the same way as anyone going through this life stage, you should take regular exercise, eat a healthy diet, aim to combat the effects of stress on your body and give up smoking to maximize your chances of a long and healthy life. Of course, just like anyone else, women of colour may not experience any symptoms at all, breezing through this stage feeling fabulous.

# The LGBTQ+ experience

It isn't only cis women who will go through perimenopause; trans women and trans men can also experience symptoms. For example, if trans women decide to lower their oestrogen intake as they get a little older, it can have the same effect as a cisgender woman experiencing the natural lowering of oestrogen levels. The advice throughout this book is still relevant for you. But if you are part of the LGBTQ+ community, following the advice to look after your heart is perhaps even more important as there may be more factors to consider that are linked to your well-being or stress levels, which would put anyone at higher risk of cardiovascular problems. Most importantly, don't be afraid to ask for support with your symptoms – from friends and your community; you need it just as much as everyone else.

# Perimenopause in different cultures

While perimenopause and menopause are universal, the way we approach them varies enormously from one culture to another. The word menopause is derived from Ancient Greek: *men*, meaning "month", and *pausis*, meaning "cessation" – so menopause simply refers to the cessation of our monthly bleed. For women in Western cultures that arguably venerate youth and beauty, perimenopause can feel like heading to the end of the road, rather than to a new beginning, and many report more severe experiences of perimenopause and menopause than in other cultures.

In Japan, *konenki* – menopause – is considered to span roughly 20 years, from around age 40 to 60. The term translates as "season of rebirth and regeneration" or "renewal of life and energy", so in Japanese, perimenopause and menopause carry positive connotations as a time of transformative change, rather than simply an ending. Japanese women report fewer negative experiences of menopause. For Mayan women, it's a time to look forward to, endowing them with greater esteem and status within the community. Known as the "second spring", it's embraced as a time of purpose, growth and new potential. This is shared across many Indigenous cultures, in which postmenopausal women are looked up to as wise women and conferred raised status, becoming community leaders. In shamanic traditions, a woman who has stopped menstruating keeps her wise blood instead of giving energy to creating potential new life. In Ayurveda, it's considered a time of "soul development" and entering elderhood.

Varying cultural attitudes to perimenopause and menopause, as well as other lifestyle and dietary factors, may play a surprisingly significant role in a woman's experience of this life stage, but we can, of course, all choose to adopt the Japanese *konenki* philosophy and see it as a season of regeneration. If we can keep the feeling that we're becoming stronger, wiser women – not just ending our fertility – perhaps some of those irksome symptoms might feel a little more bearable. So prepare to transform into a new, empowered, even more marvellous you!

# Body changes

### *Skin*

As our hormones start to drop, another common symptom we might notice is our skin losing suppleness or becoming dry, dull or itchy. But don't worry; all this needs is some self-care and a little attention to our diet to make sure we're consuming the correct nutrients. We look at this in a little more detail on page 58.

### *Belly*

A minute on the lips, several perimenopausal years on the hips: never have truer words been spoken when it comes to the time leading up to the menopause. After the age of 40, our BMR (basal metabolic rate) slows down, which means that if we continue to consume the same number of calories, our body won't burn them as efficiently. Pesky hormones also play a part in changes to where we store fat, as lower oestrogen levels mean that your body may start to store fat, rather unhelpfully, around your belly. There are some tips and advice for how to manage weight gain later in the book (see page 54).

## Boobs

The fluctuation in progesterone levels can also affect the breasts, meaning that they could become tender – in a similar way that they might do before periods. Less oestrogen in the body also affects the breast tissue itself, making it fattier – this in turn may cause boobs to drop slightly. Exercises such as press-ups will strengthen the muscles that support the breasts and could help to defy gravity! Investing in a good supportive bra is another solution for some lift. If you're not sure of your correct size, many stores provide a measuring service to ensure the right fit, while some offer online or video call services for advice on how to measure yourself (see Further Reading).

*Remember to examine your breasts regularly for signs of lumps, bumps or any unusual changes. If you are concerned or your breasts are painful, seek advice from a medical professional.*

Getting older is a privilege and a time for us to feel proud of our cumulative experiences.

NAOMI WATTS

# Ooh, my back!

Experts are not entirely sure why joint aches and pains can occur more often as we enter the perimenopause, typically – but not always – after exercise. More than likely it is another result of the change in hormone levels. Oestrogen might offer anti-inflammatory properties, so when we don't have as much of the hormone moving around our body, then muscles and joints can become swollen and painful. The neck, shoulders, wrists and knees seem to be most affected, but other joints can also become stiff and sore. You shouldn't stop exercising, but you should incorporate extra time after you've worked out to really stretch your muscles. If you sit hunched over a desk all day, then schedule time to get up and move about. If aches, pains and stiffness occur randomly, then seek medical advice to rule out other causes, such as osteoporosis (lack of oestrogen can affect bone density), arthritis or fibromyalgia.

# Headache or migraine?

We all get the occasional headache, but did you know that women are three times as likely to suffer from migraines than men are? And if you've never had one, perimenopause can unfortunately bring them on – again, due to fluctuations in hormone levels. Whereas a headache can be irritating but possible to get rid of with a couple of painkillers, a migraine might arrive with or without a headache and can affect your daily activities. Many people find the only solution is going back to bed until it abates.

Common migraine symptoms include:

- a strong throbbing pain on one side of the head (usually, but not always, present)
- nausea and/or being sick
- feeling dizzy
- stomach pain and upset tummy
- light sensitivity or seeing flashing lights

See Chapter Three for more helpful tips on managing migraines.

# Mood swings

If you've ever suffered from PMS (premenstrual syndrome) then you'll know how hormone levels and your cycle can affect how you're feeling. The perimenopause is no different, and low mood can often strike completely out of the blue. Research suggests that we have oestrogen affecting our brain to thank for this. Some people report going to bed one evening just fine, thank you; yet when they wake up they feel tense, upset, tearful, sad or downright angry – or a combination of all of these at the same time. In the next chapter we'll take a look at how you can manage these unwelcome outbursts, but rest assured that if this does happen to you, it will not last forever. Just make sure your partner knows when to duck.

# Let's get it on. Or not?

Earlier in this chapter we talked about testosterone. Predominantly a male hormone, it's important in fuelling sex drive for everyone – and like oestrogen and progesterone, falling levels can have an impact on our libido. Combine this with the fact that lower levels of progesterone can cause the walls of the vagina to become a little dry, our mood might be low and we can become quite tired or suffer from insomnia, there's potential for the perimenopause to have a negative impact on our sex life. This is not the case for everyone, though; in fact, some report that their sex life actually improves postmenopause – finally, something to look forward to! If your desire for sexual contact does wax and wane, don't be embarrassed to talk to a health professional about it. You will certainly not be the only person going through this. There are ways to deal with it and treatments that can help, which we'll explore a little more in the following chapters.

## *Put relationships first*

Though it is important to most of us, having sex is not the only way to spend quality time with someone we love. Try not to resent yourself or your partner for not wanting sex at the moment. Hugging, holding hands, practising massage, going out for a meal, chilling out together on the couch in your PJs or simply giving your partner your full attention when they talk are all things we can do to feel close to someone. This, in turn, could help your physical relationship in the long run.

# *Fatigue*

Some women report a detectable uptick in fatigue and lethargy during perimenopause. This is relatively common and is partly due to changing hormone levels, which can lead to night sweats, which disrupt restorative sleep, which leads to tiredness... and so the cycle continues. Hormones in the thyroid can also be affected, impacting energy levels; and because the urinary tract is thinner and more easily irritated, you can find yourself waking up to visit the bathroom more often during the night, too. Resting when you can and sticking to a night-time routine wherever possible can help to deal with tiredness – as can organizing your social life more effectively (see Chapter Two).

*Other conditions, such as chronic fatigue syndrome, can make you feel utterly exhausted even when well rested, so if you're concerned about your energy levels, speak to a medical practitioner.*

# Digestive troubles?

Another symptom to be on the lookout for is issues with digestion. The drop in the key hormones oestrogen and progesterone has an effect on how food travels through your gastrointestinal tract, slowing it down. Because this digestion process takes longer, more water is reabsorbed into the bloodstream, which can cause bloating, excess wind, acid reflux, indigestion, tummy cramps and an upset stomach. Hormone changes can also affect bile, a digestive fluid produced in the liver and stored in the gallbladder. Hormone reduction means that the bile is more concentrated, which can lead to gallstones and other related issues. Other conditions, including irritable bowel syndrome (IBS), can cause similar symptoms to those described above. If you experience any digestive or bowel changes that are very troubling, such as blood in your stools or sudden weight loss, then seek medical advice as a matter of urgency.

# Common myths and misconceptions

There are many misconceptions about the changes that our bodies go through as we age. Here are five of the most popular beliefs, debunked.

### 1 Menopause doesn't begin until you're at least 50.

Perimenopause – the years leading up to menopause itself – can begin as early as our thirties or forties. Many of us may have never even heard of perimenopause before picking up this book, but hopefully reading this chapter has rectified that!

### 2 You can't get pregnant once periods become irregular.

Though your fertility is likely to decline after the age of 45, falling pregnant is still possible while you are menstruating, even if your periods are not regular. It's recommended that you continue to use birth control until you have not had any periods for a full year.

### 3    Everyone will get night sweats.

As outlined earlier, everyone's experience will differ. Some may not notice anything, aside from periods stopping, and others will experience many more symptoms – including hot flushes and night sweats.

### 4    Your body will no longer produce oestrogen.

Although hormone levels decline during perimenopause, your body will continue to produce some oestrogen postmenopause. While the ovaries no longer produce it, the adrenal glands continue to manufacture enough for your body's needs.

### 5    "The change" is something to be worried and/or embarrassed about.

Absolutely not. Half the world's population will go through this. It is simply the next stage of your life and is nothing to be fearful or ashamed about. Yes, there may be some symptoms to deal with, but deal with them you can. You need only look around at the many vibrant, outgoing 60+ year-olds to see that there is indeed life on the other side!

# Chapter Two:
## *Managing Perimenopause*

In Chapter One we considered what you might expect from perimenopause and how you may recognize it. In Chapter Two we delve a little deeper, taking a look at how you might deal with some of these symptoms – whether they are physical, mental or emotional. There are actually many things you can do yourself to manage any changes that might arise, many of which are simple, free – and even fun!

## Comparison is
## the thief of joy

To start with, the number one tip is to not compare yourself, or any symptoms you may be experiencing, to others. No two people are built in the same way, and our experience of perimenopause is no different. Some bodies will cope well with any changes thrown at them, and these could be relatively short-lived; others will definitely notice more going on! That said, while you shouldn't *compare* yourself with other people, there is something to be said for *talking* about how you are feeling. You could confide in a family member who has been through this already, a health professional or a good friend. Historically, perimenopause and menopause were things that weren't discussed openly; thankfully, this is starting to change.

# Let's talk about sex

We covered how dips in oestrogen and lower testosterone levels can impact on our sex life, affecting whether we want it at all (low libido), or if we do, how it might become uncomfortable (mind is willing, but body has other ideas). Well, perimenopause does not mean that your sex life has to be confined to the history books! If you are experiencing vaginal dryness, you might find that some extra lubrication or a targeted moisturizer can make a difference. There are several types of lubricant:

- **Water-based** – usually safe for most skin types and, if being used with a condom, can be used with both latex and non-latex styles.

- **Silicone-based** – great for sensitive skin and can be used with condoms. You should avoid using them with silicone sex toys though, as they can cause abrasions where bacteria could get trapped.

- **Oil-based** – these last the longest; there's no need for frequent re-application. However, they can increase the chance of a latex condom breaking.

- **Natural** – some people prefer products that use natural ingredients; they contain far fewer chemicals that could cause irritation.

With any new product that's going to come into contact with your skin, always read the label beforehand, as some lubricants are designed to cause sensation – also make sure to test any new product on a small area first before going all in. If you're unsure what would be best for you, ask for a confidential chat with a pharmacist or consult a medical professional.

## *Go in a different direction*
What felt great before may not at the moment, and that is perfectly fine. Experiment – either with a partner or solo – and find new ways to love each other or explore your own body. Taking control of how you deal with any changes that might be headed your way will bring an amazing feeling of empowerment, too.

# *Perimenopause and sleep*

We all know how we feel after interrupted sleep; but getting a decent night's rest is easier said than done when you might have trouble dropping off, or you're feeling hot, uncomfortable or itchy. According to the Sleep Foundation, between 39 and 47 per cent of those going through perimenopause are affected by sleep problems. The most obvious culprit here is night sweats, as the rise in body temperature can wake you, and you might find it difficult to fall back asleep. Other annoyances, such as restless legs (where the legs might feel itchy or prickly, meaning you feel the urge to move them about) are at play, too. Something else that is more common at this time is snoring, as it's thought that the lack of progesterone may relax the upper airways; this, too, can disrupt our breathing and may jolt us awake. If you become a snorer (rest assured, if you're in a relationship, your partner will let you know), there are various remedies and devices to try that can help you avoid being banished to the sofa. Ask a pharmacist for some recommendations. Being well rested will help you to deal with any other symptoms you might develop, so over the next few pages are some tips to achieve a more satisfying night.

## 1. Reduce your alcohol intake

While it may help you to nod off quickly, alcohol is a stimulant. This means it can irritate your bladder, resulting in night-time bathroom trips. It also raises your body temperature, which may worsen night sweats. The best thing to have before bed is warm milk and a banana! Both of these contain tryptophan, an amino acid that helps you sleep.

## 2. Stick to a routine

Establishing a bedtime routine is good practice, even before the perimenopausal years. Don't eat or drink spicy or acidic food too late in the evening; switch to decaf tea or coffee at least a few hours before bed; have a relaxing aromatic bath or a warm shower, then relax with a book or listen to a meditation app. No scrolling on your phone, though, as the blue light it emits will stimulate your brain – and who wants to be stressing about who's going to win *Love Island* as they drop off to sleep?! If you are unable to sleep within 20 minutes, then get up, go to a different room and carry out a peaceful activity in dim lighting; then return to bed when you feel sleepy. Limit activities in bed to sleep and sex; your brain is clever and can associate your bed with all sorts of unhelpful activities that will make sleeping even harder!

### 3. Increase exercise
Upping physical activity during the day will lead to a more restful sleep – but you should ideally avoid too much aerobic exercise right before bed.

### 4. Ditch synthetic fibres
If you are buying new bedding or nightwear, go for breathable cotton, moisture-wicking material or organic fibres, like bamboo. Synthetic fibres won't allow your skin to breathe and can make sweating or itching worse.

### 5. Let in fresh air
If it's possible where you live, sleep with your windows open to keep your temperature in check. This may sound simple to do, but it may need some extra thought if you have pets, don't want to invite in mosquitoes or you are in a noisy city. Consider investing in some simple foam earplugs

to block out traffic noise (you should still hear your morning alarm through them!) and look into fitting mesh screens to keep insects out and four-legged friends in.

## 6. Avoid napping

Tempting though it is to have a snooze when you haven't slept well the previous night, try to avoid napping during the day. While you might feel better in the short term, you won't feel tired at bedtime, and so the cycle continues. Opt instead for an early night.

*As with all things perimenopausal, if you are having severe difficulty sleeping, please seek professional help.*

# And the beauty of a woman, with passing years only grows!

AUDREY HEPBURN

# Stay hydrated

While drinking caffeine and alcohol too close to bedtime can lead to interrupted sleep, it is important to keep your fluid levels up during the day. You lose water when you sweat, so if you're getting night sweats, you'll be more prone to dehydration; this can lead to dizzy spells. And let's not forget that keeping your water levels topped up will also help reduce the appearance of dry skin. Keep a reusable water bottle handy when you're working or when you're out and about, and remember to sip from it regularly. And if you're on a night out, alternate each glass of alcohol with a glass of water or a soft drink, avoiding those that contain a lot of sugar. Remember, too, that many foods contain water: watermelon, cucumber, pineapple, strawberries, blueberries, tomatoes, spinach and oranges are all water-rich, so make sure to get your five-a-day.

# Look after your heart

In Chapter One, we explained how your heart can be affected by perimenopause, so in preparation, you can give your heart a good head start! For example, walking instead of taking the bus, or using the stairs instead of jumping in the lift, are two simple things you can do to increase physical activity. If you smoke, try to take steps to stop, otherwise you are putting yourself at risk of heart problems as you get older. And good news for those with a sweet tooth: dark chocolate is rich in antioxidants, which are great for heart health. Other foods to eat for optimal heart health include leafy green veg, berries, whole grains, fatty fish, walnuts, almonds, tomatoes, olive oil and garlic.

# Soy you later!

Soy is a plant protein that contains phytoestrogens (known as isoflavones). Once in your body, these isoflavones can bind to your oestrogen receptors, so it is believed that increasing our intake can help some way with the drop in our oestrogen levels, counteracting some perimenopausal symptoms. It is best to steer clear of highly processed and genetically modified soy products and powders and instead opt a few times a week for things like organic tofu or soy milk, miso and edamame, as these offer more in the way of nutritional value. Everyone will process soy differently, so not all of us will see any benefit. But even if it does not do much for our potential perimenopause symptoms, soy is full of fibre, protein, antioxidants and omega-3 fatty acids and could replace some of the less healthy foods we might be consuming.

# *Keep moving!*

As we progress into our thirties and forties, though we feel no different on the inside we might find that our body no longer thanks us as willingly for that intensive run or HIIT (high-intensity interval training) workout; though while you feel able to, you should absolutely carry on with this! But if you do ever start to feel like changing your exercise regimen, there are other ways to benefit your body with less impact on your joints – and you'll still be able to get out of bed easily the next morning.

## *Yoga*

As well as keeping your muscles, joints and ligaments relaxed and supple, yoga brings great benefits for your mind and well-being. Most classes offer relaxation and meditation at the end of the session to focus on your breathing and sense of self, to reduce anxiety and stress. Some practitioners also offer menopause yoga, with specially adapted poses and extra props to ease joint aches and pains. You'll likely sleep better after practising yoga, too.

## Pilates

German fitness guru Joseph Pilates was often unwell as a child, so he dedicated his life to improving his physical strength. He believed that modern lifestyles and poor posture and breathing were largely to blame for bad health, so he developed a series of exercises to improve this; and lo, Pilates was born. Pilates is low impact and works to strengthen core muscles, improve flexibility and align the spine.

## Walking

Gentler on your joints than running, walking is one of the best all-round (and free) complete body workouts you can do. All you need is a good pair of walking shoes and appropriate clothing for the weather. You might also discover a new coffee shop on an exploration of your neighbourhood.

## Swimming

As well as minimum joint impact, swimming burns lots of calories. Per 30 minutes, front crawl or backstroke works off 257 calories, breaststroke zaps 367 and (if you're feeling coordinated and energetic) butterfly burns 404. (A plain sugar doughnut averages 200 calories, in case you're interested!) If you can't swim, perhaps it's time to learn; swimming exercises all the major muscle groups and is also a valuable life skill in case you ever find yourself out of your depth.

## *Aqua aerobics*

In water, around 90 per cent of your body weight is supported, so any type of activity involving $H_2O$ has to be great for your joints, plus it provides a natural resistance for your muscles. Sir Elton John revealed in an interview that he walks 6 miles (nearly 10 km) a week in his local pool, so if it's good enough for the rocket man...

## *Dance like no one is watching*

There's no reason why dancing should only happen on a dance floor; moving to music is great for the body and the soul, sending out a flood of endorphins and shaking off stress. So liven up a midweek dinnertime by cooking along to a kitchen disco! Or why not seek out a local dance class and learn to tango, waltz or cha-cha like a pro?

## *Pedal power*

Another activity that's kinder to your joints and builds muscle is cycling, either static in a gym or out in the fresh air. It's low impact, so it puts less stress on your knees, hips and feet, while the cycling movement keeps joints lubricated and moving easily. And you can choose the intensity: easier (on a flat road) or more intensive (uphill). If you're out and about, always wear a helmet!

*If you're new to exercise, consult a medical professional before you embark on a new activity – and start with something gentle, such as walking or swimming.*

# Keeping your weight in check

To reduce the chances of the dreaded middle-aged spread, one of the best things you can do is increase your physical activity. But which kind of exercise is best? After the age of 30 we lose around 1 per cent of our muscle mass every year, so (doing the maths) that means nearly 10 per cent of our muscle mass has dwindled by the age of 40. For anyone – but particularly if you are over age 40 – resistance training two or three times a week is one of the best things you can do to stay trim. Lifting weights builds muscle to replace what you might be losing because of lower hormone levels; it will also help to increase bone mass to stave off osteoporosis – so it's a win–win. At least to begin with, it's worth taking a class or seeking some advice from a pro to learn the correct technique and reduce the risk of injury. You don't have to go full Popeye and pump iron and hoist barbells in the gym. Kettlebell classes are growing in popularity and are a really fun way to burn calories while lifting weights to music, and some yoga and Pilates instructors incorporate weights or resistance bands into their classes to help you tone up. Increasing your cardio activity (walking more, driving less) in combination with resistance training means you'll be getting a total body workout as well as reducing your carbon footprint.

*If you haven't been very physically active in the past, start slowly and consult a health professional before embarking on any new exercise regimen.*

*Always warm up beforehand to prevent injury, and remember to stretch after any workout; your muscles will thank you the next day!*

# Every cloud has a silver lining

Now you have reached the halfway point of the book, you might be starting to think there's a lot more to this perimenopause than you thought. But don't despair; there's absolutely no reason to worry about any changes that might come your way. In Chapter Three, we outline some of the support available for perimenopausal symptoms, should you feel you need it. But in the meantime, staying positive is the best way to deal with any changes. Why not try starting a gratitude journal and writing in it every evening? Make a note of three things you are thankful for that day, about yourself and your life. This could be fabulous friends, a loving family or partner, a job you enjoy, good health, somewhere comfortable and safe to live – or even that amazing espresso that kept you awake through a presentation at work.

# LOL!

One of the most excellent ways to lift a bad mood is to have a good old-fashioned "stop it, I can't breathe" belly laugh. Laughter not only gives your heart and diaphragm a great workout, but also releases endorphins and lowers cortisol levels, giving you an amazing physical release of stress. Also, rather fascinatingly, it makes our T cells (which are responsible for propping up our immune system) more effective. Research has also shown that even fake laughter has the same effect. So next time you're in need of a pick-me-up, put your favourite funny film or comedy show on TV, check out a live local comedian at an open mic night or just have a good old gossip with your besties. Laughter really is the best medicine.

*Laughter therapy is an actual thing! Check out laughternetwork.wordpress.com.*

# *Feel-good vitamins and minerals*

Ice cream aside (there is *always* an allowance for the odd treat), the kind of food that we put into our mouth should support our body in how it deals with the changes that might be in store. Certain vitamins become more useful as we head into perimenopause, so on the next four pages is a rundown of what you might need more of, and where to get it.

*Remember, while it's usually better to get your vitamins from natural sources, supplements are there to assist when you're run down, have a particular food allergy or sensitivity or can't get enough from your diet – perhaps due to seasonal availability.*

## *Vitamin D*
Vitamin D is known as the sunshine vitamin, as your body produces it after exposure to daylight; ideally we should all spend at least 15 minutes

outside each day. During the darker months, a supplement is useful. Vitamin D deficiency could increase your risk of fractures and lead to softening of bones. As well as daylight, you get it from fatty fish, cheese, mushrooms, fortified cereals and orange juice, and egg yolks. The recommended dose is 15 mcg per day, or 20 mcg per day if you are over 50.

## *Two B, or not two B*

The two essential B vitamins are B6 and B12. They have different roles to play in the body. B6 helps in the production of serotonin, a chemical that helps to keep our emotions stable. As we get older, our levels of B6 can drop, which might explain those perimenopausal mood swings! Aim for 1.3 mg per day. B12 is good for bone and brain health. It is water soluble and found in a lot of foods including sardines, milk and meat; it is often also added to things like breakfast cereals. Again, as we get older our body can't absorb it as easily, so we need to top it up to avoid becoming deficient. Signs of low levels of B12 include fatigue, loss of appetite and dizziness. The recommended intake of B12 is 2.4 mg per day.

*If you have existing health issues, including kidney problems, high blood pressure or gastrointestinal issues, consult a health professional before taking extra vitamins.*

## Magnesium

Good sources of magnesium (recommended amount 310 mg per day) include dark chocolate, dark leafy greens, cashews, peanut butter, tofu and salmon. As well as helping to maintain nerves and muscles and support brain health, this impressive all-rounder takes care of your bones and teeth. It also boosts your metabolism, reducing fatigue. Magnesium assists with moving electrolytes into cells, regulating your heartbeat and controlling palpitations (so you can watch those Chris Hemsworth movies to your heart's content!).

## Vitamin E

Many perimenopausal symptoms can lead to stress, which leads to cell damage, which in turn increases your risk of weight gain, heart disease and low mood. Vitamin E is an antioxidant that helps to fight cell damage and might also lower inflammation in the body. Good sources of the recommended 15 mg a day are almonds, avocados, shellfish and wheatgerm.

# A quick vitamin pick-me-up

*(Serves 1)*

As mentioned on page 43, bananas are great for helping you sleep. Combined with the other ingredients here, they'll provide a fabulous burst of vitamins.

### *Ingredients*

- 200 ml almond or oat milk
- 1 ripe banana
- 6 chunks fresh pineapple
- 1 tablespoon milled flaxseed mix (optional)
- 1 teaspoon honey or ½ teaspoon vanilla extract for a touch of sweetness (optional)

### *Method*

Pop it all into a blender, whizz together, pour into a glass and enjoy.

# Food and sex

No, this is not what you think! Did you know certain foods might help to boost your libido?

*Pineapples* – As well as being packed with vitamins and antioxidants, pineapple can regulate hormones. This super-fruit, which contains an enzyme called bromelain, can increase testosterone production, which, as we saw earlier in the book, affects libido. It can also help to regulate serotonin levels.

*Pumpkin seeds and pine nuts* – These are both a fantastic source of testosterone-boosting zinc, as well as lots of other things that are good for you. Sprinkle them all over a salad, or enjoy a bowl of pasta with fresh pesto, which is made with pine nuts. Yum!

*Red grapes* – Red grapes contain boron, a mineral that can boost the production of both oestrogen and testosterone. A handful of grapes will satisfy those evening sugar cravings, too.

*Strawberries* – Strawberries are packed with folic acid, omega-3 fatty acids and Vitamin C, all of which boost sex drive and increase blood flow around the body.

*Sweet potatoes* – These tasty carbs are chock-full of Vitamin A, beta carotene, potassium and antioxidants, all of which could kick-start a flagging sex drive.

*Asparagus* – This tasty veg supplies you with plenty of sex-hormone-producing potassium, and many other vitamins and goodies, including an amino acid called asparagine, which is important for brain health. It also cleans the urinary tract, which is why your urine can look and smell a bit interesting the next day!

*Walnuts and kidney beans* – These two beauties contain a substance called L-arginine. This is converted into nitric oxide in the body, dilating blood vessels and increasing blood flow. Need we say more?

# Perimenopause at work

Almost half of the global workforce will go through the menopause, so if you're affected by symptoms at work and feel like you're the only one, then you probably aren't! When it comes to experiencing symptoms at work, many of us tend to try and suck it up. But suffering in silence could actually affect your career – in fact, in one study of 4,000 women, 85 per cent said they had no one at work to talk to about their symptoms, and 10 per cent had left their jobs because of this. Chat to your colleagues if you work in the sort of environment where this is acceptable, and if you feel comfortable doing so; but at the very least, you should have a conversation with your manager or human resources or occupational health departments to explain how your symptoms are affecting your work. It might be a good idea to suggest any solutions you have in mind to open the discussion – for example, having a desk fan. Historically, talking about the menopause has been taboo, but in many countries this is finally beginning to change. Some companies are even introducing menopause policies outlining specific support available. If your workplace doesn't have one yet, then perhaps you can be the catalyst.

## *Working solo*

On the flip side of being caught out by a hot flush in the office, many of us now spend more time working remotely. Hot flushes, brain fog and anxiety can strike via Zoom, too! You might not want to have your camera switched on as you feel under scrutiny or uncomfortable, and that's fine. The same advice applies: talk to your manager or your colleagues about how you're feeling. It shouldn't be the end of the world if you sometimes need to be on audio only.

# How to manage a drop in energy levels

This may sound obvious, but if you find yourself lacking in energy, accept it and be kind to yourself. If you need to cancel plans as you can't face being sociable, or you need to take time to just chill out on the sofa after a busy day, that's OK. With fluctuating hormones and interrupted sleep, perimenopause can be pretty tiring – and it might be enough to simply stay upright until bedtime. There may be some weeks where you may feel like you could rule the world, and other mornings you can barely summon the energy to put on socks. This is – and it can't be said enough – completely normal. Again, as with any other symptom, tiredness won't affect everyone in the same way, if at all. So turn off the TV, brew a camomile tea and have an early night. Tomorrow is another day.

# Dealing with anxious thoughts

As mentioned in Chapter One, feeling anxious can often become more common during perimenopause. Although this is likely to be temporary, if you are normally really outgoing it can take you by surprise. If you're feeling nervous about an approaching social event, a presentation you need to give at work or a date with someone new, for example, try some deep breathing using the 4–7–8 technique. Lie down somewhere quiet, breathe in deeply for 4 seconds, hold your breath for 7 seconds, then exhale slowly for a count of 8 seconds. Aim to do this for 15 minutes if you can. Regular endorphin-boosting exercise, getting enough rest and maintaining a positive attitude will also help you cope better with any worries if they come along. If it really comes to it, cancel or rearrange any plans; your mental health is more important.

# Be aware of sugar cravings

Some research has shown that in the lead-up to menopause, our bodies don't burn as many calories because our metabolic rate starts to slow – but feeling tired can often mean that our body craves sugar to keep going. It's important therefore during perimenopause, when this slowing metabolism means we are prone to weight gain, to limit refined sugar – like that found in biscuits and sweets. Be aware also of hidden sugar added to food you might not expect, like sliced bread, so check the labels when you're shopping. Eating a balanced diet rich in vital vitamins and nutrients (see page 58) and drinking enough water could help you to control the urge to snack; if your stomach is full, you might not actually feel the need.

## *Swapping sugar for other snacks*

If you're a post-dinner snacker, try changing into your pyjamas after you've eaten your evening meal. Psychologically, your brain will prepare itself for bed, so you're less likely to keep eating. And if you associate snacking with watching TV, mix it up and listen to a podcast or read a book. But let's face it, we're all human; if you really do need to give in to the craving, replace a chocolate bar or bag of crisps with a handful of plain cashew nuts with raisins, some strawberries, grapes or a banana, and swap an alcoholic nightcap with a cup of decaffeinated or herbal tea.

*Don't expect to beat your snack cravings instantly; it takes time to break an established habit. The best way is to replace an old behaviour with a new, healthier one – which, with repetition, will soon become habitual.*

## Timing is everything

Did you know that the optimum time between an evening meal and breakfast the next day is 12 hours? Giving your digestive system a break allows it to, in effect, carry out essential maintenance and boost your immune system. And without excess food to digest, your body is more likely to burn fat.

# Oral health

This may not be a symptom you've heard of, but a drop in oestrogen levels during perimenopause can lead to potential dental issues. Loss of bone density can affect the jaw in the same way as other parts of the body, resulting in tooth problems. Keep on top of your dental hygiene by brushing twice a day and flossing regularly – you may prefer to use a rechargeable electric toothbrush rather than a manual one for optimum plaque removal. Keep a look out, too, for any kind of gum issues: swollen or red gums, bleeding after brushing or tenderness. And in the same way that other areas can experience dryness, so too can your mouth. If you don't produce enough saliva to wash them away, germs and bacteria can multiply. Visit a dentist regularly, so any issues are caught early on and nipped in the bud.

I'm baffled that anyone might not think women get more beautiful as they get older.

**KATE WINSLET**

# Love your gut

In Chapter One, we outlined how perimenopause can disrupt your digestive system. The best way to deal with any potential issues is by giving your gut a little TLC, starting now! Eating a healthy, balanced diet full of whole grains, fresh fruit and veg, as well as limiting your alcohol intake, will make you feel your best; but here are a few more pointers to keep your insides in tip-top condition.

## *Probiotics*

There is some evidence that taking probiotics (live or "friendly" bacteria) can help to stabilize your tummy and bowel during perimenopause by stimulating your body to produce the necessary mucus. They may also help with the dreaded hot flushes. Probiotics are added to many foods, including yogurt, pickles, sauerkraut, sourdough bread and some types of cheese. Supplements are also available, but speak to a medical professional or pharmacist for advice about these.

## *Slow down*

If you are affected by morning stomach trouble, take a little extra time to let your body wake up and your hormones to settle before eating breakfast. And when you do eat, make sure it's a balanced meal consisting of as little processed food as possible, accompanied by a glass of water to help it move more easily through your system. Chew your food thoroughly, too, as this means your body doesn't have to work as hard to digest it. Cutting down on sugar and caffeine can also give your tummy a rest if you're feeling overloaded.

## Beat the bloat

If you suffer with excess gas or bloating, then peppermint, turmeric or ginger tea can work wonders. For constipation, try increasing the amount of fibre in your diet. Be sure to do this gradually, though, or you might find you create a different problem.

*Find it hard to stomach an actual meal first thing in the morning? Try a breakfast smoothie including probiotic yogurt, oats and fruit. Kiwis and plums, in particular, are useful for keeping you regular.*

# Look after your bones

Many of us might pay little attention to our bones until they start to cause us problems, so it's vital that we do as much as possible to keep our inner structure strong and healthy. As we get older we lose bone density, which can lead to us fracturing and breaking bones more easily (osteoporosis). Females are more at risk of osteoporosis as, generally (though not always), they have smaller bones and a longer life expectancy; so they have to keep going for longer! Smoking and drinking too much alcohol can also be risk factors for weaker bones as we get older.

## *A strong foundation*

So then, what *should* we be doing for optimum bone health? Getting the right vitamins is an important factor (see page 58), as is consuming enough calcium; 700 mg per day for most adults is recommended. If we don't take in enough calcium, then our body will steal it from our bones as it is also needed for our blood to clot and to keep our heart healthy, our muscles strong and our teeth in our gums. Good sources of calcium are milk, cheese, yogurt, tinned fish, almonds, fortified bread, kale and broccoli (be careful not to boil broccoli to death, though, as you will kill all the nutrients).

## Swap TV for training

Staying active will keep your skeleton in excellent condition for years to come, so ditch that sedentary lifestyle! Weight-bearing activities in particular are good for you as you get into your thirties and forties – think dancing, hill-walking, skipping or even gardening. Anything you can do to keep moving will be of benefit. See pages 50–53 for lots of general exercise tips to keep you fit and healthy.

# Skin deep

To add some glow to a dull complexion, try one of these homemade face rejuvenators. Test a little on a small area, such as your wrist or behind your ear, 24 hours beforehand, in case you react to any of the ingredients.

## Avocado and oat face mask

Blitz 1 tablespoon rolled oats in a food processor and tip into a bowl. Add 120 g avocado, 1 teaspoon fresh lemon juice, 2 teaspoons honey and 2 teaspoons coconut oil. Mush together to a smooth consistency. Apply to a clean, dry face for 15 minutes, then remove with warm water and a face cloth. Avocado is great for hydrating, oats exfoliate and nourish, lemon cleanses, and honey and coconut oil are antibacterial and moisturizing.

## Yogurt and honey face mask

The lactic acid in yogurt will bring some oomph to your complexion by sloughing off old skin cells, while honey will restore moisture and elasticity. Combine a dollop of natural yogurt with 1 tablespoon clear honey; mix together and apply. After 10 minutes, rinse with warm water.

Gravity and wrinkles are fine with me. They're a small price to pay for the new wisdom inside my head and my heart.

**DREW BARRYMORE**

# Be mindful

Mindfulness is the ability to be fully present in the moment, to enjoy and take pleasure in just being in the here and now. Practising mindfulness regularly can bring about a reduction in stress, allowing you to become calmer and more centred and focused. In turn, you'll be better able to deal with any possible side effects that you might encounter as a result of perimenopause, such as anxiety and brain fog. There are many ways to build mindfulness into your daily life. We have already mentioned that chewing your food more slowly will allow your body to digest it more easily, but why not take this one step further and practise *mindful* eating? This means paying complete attention to your meals, with no distractions, rather than stuffing it down as quickly as you can so you can binge-watch your favourite shows! Really engage all five of your senses every time you eat, savouring the taste, smell and texture of your food. Using your eyes and brain in conjunction with your stomach will also give your body time to establish whether it's full, which means you might not actually "need" that sugary treat.

Other ways to practise daily mindfulness include actively listening to other people when they are speaking to you – this means using your ears to hear them and your eyes to look at them. If you are able to really hone your listening skills, then your conversations will become more meaningful and people will be more likely to pay attention to you if you ever need to discuss anything – menopause-related or otherwise! You can also practise mindfulness when you are out and about. Rather than wandering along the street checking your phone messages, pay attention to what is going on around you; listen to beautiful birdsong, feel the warm sunshine on your face, hear the wind whispering through the trees.

# Looking after your mental health

The emotional and psychological symptoms you might encounter during perimenopause can arise in several forms, from anxiety and depression to brain fog and mood swings. Knowing that they will pass and actually going through them are two quite different things, however. If you're worried about any symptoms you experience, please do talk to someone, whether it's a close friend, your partner or a professional. If you need a day off work, ask for one. If you can't face the weekly grocery shop, order online. Simply doing something you really enjoy instead of boring chores can bring equilibrium to your headspace as well. Bake a cake rather than vacuum; who's going to notice a little dust when you are offering them a slice of lemon drizzle?

*Keep a countdown on your phone that counts down to events you're looking forward to. Try to find something you enjoy every day, and celebrate little wins.*

It's a time of liberation... It's a time of shedding the shackles of inhibition and of giving a damn.

DAVINA McCALL
ON MENOPAUSE

# Stress busters

Just as the symptoms of perimenopause will affect us all in our own way, how we deal with them will be individual, too – many of us might find we are more stressed than usual, for example. So here is some more advice to use alongside all the other tips in this book, to keep you calm along the way.

**Balance work and home** – With many of us now working more hours in our home, it's more important than ever to make that separation between work and home life. Try leaving the house when you are done with work and "coming home" through the front door to replicate the commute and help your brain to switch gears.

**Get outdoors** – Practise the Japanese art of *shinrin-yoku* (forest bathing; see the Further Reading section) or simply walk barefoot in the grass or go for a walk in the rain. Puddle-jumping is not just for toddlers.

**Spend time with pets** – Many studies have shown that spending time with animals can lower our stress levels by as much as half. If you don't have pets, borrow someone else's or visit a local animal park.

*Take up a hobby* – Make more time to do the things you love, whether that's crocheting, baking, reading or driving monster trucks. Doing things that make us happy is a definitive way to release endorphins and lower those cortisol levels!

*Better out than in* – If you've had a rubbish day, scream, shout, let it all out! Traditional Chinese medicine links emotions directly to health, and followers believe that shouting is great for the health of your lungs (which are linked to sadness) and liver (linked to anger and irritability). It's probably best, though, to direct your frustration into a pillow rather than at a fellow human.

*Persistent stress can negatively affect your well-being, so if you begin to feel that nothing is helping with your stress levels, do seek professional help.*

# *Take charge of your social diary*

We've all had that social invite that we feel obliged to accept, haven't we? If you are one of the lucky ones who can be honest from the outset and say you're not feeling up to it, then well done you! But for most of us, feelings of guilt creep in and we feel obliged to say yes; so on Friday night, there we are, drink in hand, pretending to have a good time. It really is OK – empowering, even – to say "no". You will do yourself no favours by overdoing it. If you've had something in the diary for a while and can't duck out completely, then make an excuse and exit early. Sometimes what your body and mind need is simply to rest and reset. So be attuned to your body's cues when it's time to take it easy – far better to manage your social life to suit your needs than to let it rule you.

# We're looking at ageing as a bad thing, but if you're doing it, you are really lucky.

**CAMERON DIAZ**

# *Track your symptoms*

Keeping a symptom diary is an excellent way to track anything that you might be experiencing; this will also come in handy if you decide to consult a medical professional. Jot notes in your phone, keep pen and paper by your bed or use sticky notes on the fridge. There are also lots of trackers available online that you can download and print: search for "menopause symptom tracker". Each day, make a note of any symptoms or changes and their severity – perhaps by giving them a rating from one to ten – as well as anything you did to deal with them; remember to note positive observations, too. As we've stated throughout this book so far, everyone's journey through, and experience of, perimenopause will be completely personal to them; but if you are interested in finding out what treatments are available to help, then check out Chapter Three.

# Celebrate you!

As stated at the very start of the book, you may sail blissfully through this phase of life and notice very little change at all. If you do start to notice changes, though, then following the advice and tips throughout the first two chapters of this book – and seeking help, support and advice if you need it (see Chapter Three) – means you'll be able to cope with whatever perimenopause might fling at you. So chillax, reduce your stress, eat well and exercise regularly – however that looks for you – and surround yourself with your tribe. Above all, celebrate yourself for who you are, flaws and all. Look in the mirror each day and tell yourself (out loud) that you are fabulous! And remember, nobody is perfect; even supposedly perfect celebrities enjoy the occasional pizza.

Invest in your brain, invest in your talents. Those things can appreciate and they get better as you get older.

**RASHIDA JONES**

# Chapter Three:
## *Seeking Support and Treatments*

Having now found out what perimenopause is, why it happens, how it might affect you and some of the symptoms you might expect, this chapter moves on to look at available treatments – should you wish to go down that route – and offers some advice and support. Treatments aren't just purely medical; there are lots of other things we can do to help ourselves along the road to postmenopausal marvellousness!

# When and how to seek help

## *When?*

There is absolutely no shame in asking for help if you need it along your journey through perimenopause. What form this help might take and how it can be accessed will be found throughout this chapter – including self-help, alternative and holistic therapies, or medical intervention. Many people prefer to, can, and do manage their symptoms very successfully themselves. However, if you feel that your ability to function day-to-day is being affected, your general well-being is suffering, your relationships are under strain (this can be a testing time for partners, too), brain fog is impacting your job or stress is affecting your mental health, then it might be time to seek out some professional assistance. It takes strength to ask for help, but there is no need to suffer in silence.

## *How?*

The best port of call to start with is probably a medical professional. Remember, all women are going to go through this at some point, so don't be ashamed about talking to someone; they really have seen and heard it all before. To help, take your symptom tracker (outlined in Chapter Two) and make extra notes to refer to if you need them. Begin by explaining why you are there, what symptoms or changes you are experiencing and how they are affecting you. One of the main medical treatments you might be offered for perimenopause symptoms is HRT; there is an outline of what this does, the different forms it takes, along with benefits and risks, on the following pages.

# Hormone Replacement Therapy (HRT)

The decision to take HRT is one only you can make, in consultation with a health professional. To help you decide if it might be right for you, here are some facts.

*What does HRT do?* – HRT replaces the hormones that your body begins to lose – namely, oestrogen and progesterone. It is most effective when given during perimenopause before any symptoms worsen. You can be prescribed both hormones together (combined HRT), or if you no longer have a womb or use an IUD (intrauterine device, or a coil), then you may just be offered oestrogen.

*What form does it take?* – Progesterone is usually given as a tablet, or as an IUD/coil. IUDs are usually replaced every four to five years. Oestrogen is given as pills, creams, sprays or skin patches.

*Are there any side effects?* – Initial side effects include bleeding and breast tenderness, although these usually ease within the first few months.

*Are there any risks?* – Taking oestrogen alone can thicken the lining of the womb and increase the risk of uterine cancer, so progesterone is given at the same time to counteract this risk. It is thought that combined HRT carries a small risk of breast cancer; however, this is considered lower than the risk of breast cancer if you are obese or drink moderate amounts of alcohol. Recent research outlines that the benefits of HRT outweigh the risks. Any risk will vary from person to person, so these are always best discussed with your health professional.

*What are the benefits?* – HRT can relieve most symptoms effectively. It also protects against loss of bone density. Most people who take it can notice an improvement within three to six months. HRT can also protect against the risk of heart disease or stroke: oestrogen helps to keep your cholesterol in check and protects the artery walls from fatty deposits.

*There are other medications that can be prescribed. A health professional can talk through your options with you.*

# Solutions to vaginal dryness

Many people are embarrassed to discuss vaginal dryness with a medical professional. While this is understandable – it's not the easiest subject to broach – the symptom isn't something that you should put up with. As well as affecting your sex life, it can become generally very uncomfortable and impact your daily life. If you find it a difficult subject to talk about, then speaking to a health professional of the same gender as you may help. Oestrogen creams, gels, rings and pessaries that can be used directly in the vagina can assist with symptoms; these are generally considered low risk and target the affected area directly. Or you might consider an over-the-counter lubricant or moisturizer (see pages 40–41). Another thing to think about is using sanitary pads, liners or period pants, rather than tampons – and try not to scratch, as this can exacerbate the issue.

# *What about antidepressants?*

As explained in Chapter One, fluctuating hormones can lead to low mood; research has shown that more than 50 per cent of people are affected in this way. You may be offered antidepressants when you first visit a medical professional but, though this may eventually be the correct plan of action for you, it isn't generally recommended as a first plan of action, as it is thought that it is better to deal with the cause of the low mood itself – that is, the low hormone levels. That being said, some antidepressants, such as citalopram or venlafaxine, can be used in small doses to effectively treat hot flushes in people who are unable to take HRT. If you are feeling down, make sure to eat a healthy, balanced diet full of the right vitamins and minerals, along with taking plenty of exercise and getting rest when you need it.

# How to communicate your needs

There is often nothing more therapeutic than talking about what you're going through with the people who love you. A caring partner, a great friend or understanding housemate should be able to listen to what you need and take it on board. Though they may not be going through the same thing, by explaining to them how you feel and what you're going through, they might be better prepared to help you along your journey and give you the support that you require. Don't blurt it all out in a rage, though, when you've yet again tripped over their shoes in the hallway! Choose a time when you're feeling relaxed, make a cup of tea or pour a glass of wine and settle down for a good chat. If it turns out they're going through the perimenopause, too, then you've both found someone to confide in.

## *Ask your partner to read this next bit...*

- Read this book to learn more about perimenopause and how it's affecting your partner so you will be in a stronger position to try and understand what they're going through.

- Accept that sometimes they will be grumpy/worried/anxious/tired/subdued. This is not normally anything to do with you, and much more to do with their changing balance of hormones. Try not to take it personally, but do offer to help – with chores, for example, or a sympathetic ear; just listening will be a huge support.

- Aim to not let things escalate when cross words might be exchanged. In this case, it is best to walk away.

- Remember that some of the symptoms your partner might be experiencing affect their appearance, and therefore often their self-esteem. They are still the same person you fell in love with, so let them know. Sex is not the only way to do this; very often all you might need to do is bring them a coffee and a chocolate doughnut.

# Seek support

If you don't have a partner or people in your life you can talk things through with, then counselling and support groups could offer you the sounding board that you need. There are a plethora of forums and support groups online where you can talk through anything and everything with other people going through the same as you; in particular, the "Shhh Menopause Collective" on Facebook has a thriving discussion community, and "Balance Menopause" posts lots of useful information and hosts live Q&A sessions. More formal counselling might help you to unravel the cause of your symptoms and aid you in building your self-confidence and self-esteem if these have been affected. Depending on where you live, you might need to be referred to a counsellor, so visit a health professional as your first stop.

# *Learn to love your changing body*

While perimenopause means that your body might be going through a few alterations on the outside, possibly resulting in a few more wobbly bits and some obvious wrinkles (or laughter lines, as we prefer to call them), remember you are the same person on the inside. It can be natural to feel a little out of kilter if you can no longer slide your legs into your skinny jeans without a little effort, or you don't fill your animal print bikini in quite the same way. But then again, who cares?! As many wise women have said, the best way to get a bikini body is to "buy a bikini and put it on your body". If you would feel more comfortable losing a few pounds, though, turn to page 54 for some advice on how best to control your weight during perimenopause.

# Managing migraines

We covered the symptoms of migraines in Chapter One, so if you are already familiar with them and notice an increase, or start to suffer when you haven't before, here are some tips on how to treat them.

- Learning to recognize your symptoms means you might be able to catch a migraine early so it does not become a fully-fledged headbanger. If you feel one coming on, then head for bed with an eye mask, or lie down in a dark room.

- Some people find that paracetamol, aspirin or ibuprofen will deal with them, whereas others may need medicines containing a stronger painkiller. Some of these are available over the counter, whereas some might need to be prescribed by a medical professional as they are not suitable for everyone. Triptans can replicate serotonin and calm the pain nerves, while anti-emetics tackle feelings of nausea and being sick.

- If you prefer not to, or cannot, take painkillers, then a cutaneous headache stick (usually containing menthol) or a cooling gel patch may help to relax your temples and alleviate any pain.

- One study showed that increasing magnesium in your diet can help to prevent some types of migraine, so be sure to eat a variety of nuts as this is a great source. Magnesium also offers many other benefits during perimenopause – see page 60.

- As well as stress and tiredness, certain food and drink can trigger migraines (cheese, chocolate, alcohol, too much caffeine, monosodium glutamate (MSG) or sweeteners are often to blame), so keeping a food diary to see if you can identify a culprit might help to limit them.

# Do you like it cold?

Calling all adrenaline seekers! There is more and more evidence emerging that cold water or wild swimming can do wonders for perimenopause symptoms, with many participants extolling the benefits of spending time in the sea, lakes or outdoor freshwater pools. As well as seeming to reset internal body temperature, lowering the occurrence of hot flushes, it also appears to help improve migraines and boost the immune system. Open-water swimmers report that they feel reset, happy and rejuvenated and have had their anxiety and stiff joints eased from connecting with nature in this way.

*Take part safely by joining an organized group rather than going alone and stay close to the edge, keeping aware of any tides or currents. Many open-water swimmers use a swim buoy for visibility and safety. Remember not to go swimming in cold water during extremely hot weather, and conversely, leave the water for dry land to warm up.*

# Massage

Massage is an excellent way to soothe away any perimenopause-induced aches, pains and stress, improving your overall well-being. If you have a willing partner, get them involved; this can be a lovely way to be intimate with each other. Essential oils like rose, cypress and geranium can help with hormone regulation, and if you are being bothered by hot flushes, then peppermint or lemon can help with this. To improve mood, try bergamot, neroli or jasmine, and to help you sleep, sprinkle a little lavender oil on your pillowcase. Visiting a professional masseuse is also an amazing escape, allowing you to concentrate on just you and your needs. Do take care with massage if you are pregnant, or trying to be, as some types of massage and some oils – such as camomile, clary sage and jasmine – are not suitable. In this case, it is probably best to visit a pro.

# Menopause gets a really bad rap and needs a bit of rebranding.

**GWYNETH PALTROW**

# *Herbal supplements*

Taken in tandem with a healthy lifestyle, there are several herbal supplements that you can try in order to treat symptoms such as night sweats, hot flushes and low mood. The one you might have heard of is St John's Wort, which is thought to increase serotonin in the body. It can interfere with other medications (including some forms of contraception), so do consult your health professional first if you are thinking of taking it. Other popular supplements include black cohosh to regulate hormones (not recommended for those with liver disease); agnus-castus to stabilize your moods; evening primrose oil for hot flushes; red ginseng to increase desire; and soya and red clover – both containing plant phytoestrogens – to help reduce sweating. Always read the label before you take any kind of supplement, as some need to be taken with food, and some without – and be sure to buy supplements from a reputable pharmacist.

# Mind over matter

If you would prefer not to go down a traditional medical route of dealing with perimenopause symptoms, then perhaps you could consider Cognitive Behavioural Therapy (CBT) or Neuro-Linguistic Programming (NLP). Let's look at each of these in turn.

## *Cognitive Behavioural Therapy*

CBT is a talking therapy, which reframes how you might look at your symptoms by changing the way you think and respond. Its traditional use is for depression and anxiety (both linked to perimenopause), though it can be used to address a host of other issues. It makes a link between how you feel and your physical being, asking you to focus on helpful rather than unhelpful thought processes so that you don't get caught in a vicious cycle that feels difficult to break out of. It isn't a cure, but rather an outlet to enable you to better cope. A typical CBT session involves working with a therapist to look at your problems; they will work to support you with strategies to better manage unhelpful thoughts or patterns of behaviour with the aim of you integrating these new coping strategies into your day-to-day life.

## *Neuro-Linguistic Programming*

NLP has been around since the 1970s, when it was started in the US by psychology student, Richard Bandler, and John Grinder, a professor of linguistics. But what is it, and how can it help with perimenopause? NLP is essentially the study of how we can help ourselves to focus on solutions rather than problems. It focuses on our body language, as well as *how* we talk and the language we use. For example, don't catch a glimpse of yourself, droopy shouldered in a mirror, and think, "Gosh, I look really old and tired". Reframe it as, "If I get an early night, I'll feel much better tomorrow". Rather than focusing on how any symptoms are interfering with your life, think about how you can best deal with them. The more you do this, the more it will come naturally to you, increasing your positive vibes.

# Hypnotherapy

Traditional hypnosis often conjures images of magicians on stage putting people into a trance and then asking them to act like chickens. Well, there is much more to it than that. Clinical hypnotherapy can teach you a range of self-hypnosis techniques to employ calming imagery when symptoms arise – for example, imagining that you are stepping into cooling water or feeling a cold breeze blowing through your hair to alleviate sweating. In one particular study, 200 women reported 74 per cent fewer hot flushes after five 45-minute sessions, as well as a general improvement in sleep. There is no loss of control during a hypnotherapy session; it is similar in many ways to meditation, closing out intrusive thoughts and distractions to enter a state of relaxation and peace, and ultimately being brought back to full awareness.

# Acupuncture

Acupuncture is an alternative therapy used in traditional Chinese medicine that carries very few side effects. It involves the insertion of very thin needles into pressure points in the connective tissue – or fascia – in the body to restore the flow of energy. The aim of this is to promote healing and reduce stress by stimulating the production of serotonin and endorphins in the brain. One small study found that receiving regular acupuncture over five weeks reduced sleep problems, hot flushes, sweats and mood swings, while another found that it can alter neurotransmitters in the brain and improve mood. A qualified acupuncturist should spend time talking to you at an initial consultation about why you are there and what you hope to achieve.

# *Reflexology*

This restorative and relaxing ancient therapy for body and mind focuses on applying pressure to areas on the soles of the feet (and sometimes points on the hands) to identify imbalances and stimulate healing. It works by linking the areas on the feet or hands to corresponding areas in the body via energy connections, or channels. It is thought that stress can block these energy channels, so a qualified reflexologist works on unblocking them, getting the energy flowing and promoting renewal. Reflexology has been known to benefit and treat things such as migraine, urinary tract and digestion issues, anxiety and hormone imbalances – in other words, many of the symptoms of perimenopause! During a session you might experience sensations of tingling or warmth, and some people do report side effects including nausea and feeling light-headed. People with certain conditions like gout or circulatory issues, or who have foot injuries, might not be suited to reflexology, though, so if you are unsure do consult a health professional first.

# *Foot Reflexology Chart*

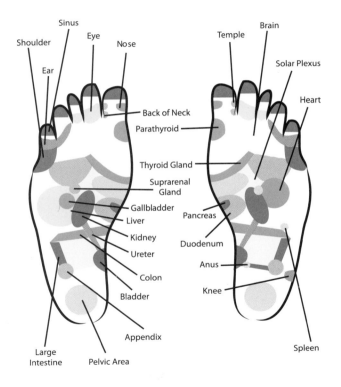

Sinus
Shoulder
Eye
Nose
Ear
Temple
Brain
Solar Plexus
Heart
Back of Neck
Parathyroid
Thyroid Gland
Suprarenal Gland
Gallbladder
Liver
Kidney
Ureter
Colon
Bladder
Pancreas
Duodenum
Anus
Knee
Appendix
Large Intestine
Pelvic Area
Spleen

# Reiki

Reiki is a gentle but powerful complimentary therapy with origins in Japan. It uses a natural and non-intrusive method of hands-on healing, with the aim of restoring balance and harmony to the mind, body and emotions. Rei (*ray*) means "the higher power", and Ki (*kee*) means "life-force energy" – it is believed that this energy flows through all living things.

## How does it work?
Reiki works by a practitioner harnessing their own life-force energy and transferring this to someone else to promote healing. Unlike massage, a patient remains fully clothed, and a Reiki practitioner holds their hands above and/or below a particular area of the body – without actually touching, or very lightly resting on, the skin.

## What are the benefits for the perimenopause?
Reiki is effective in helping symptoms of perimenopause and menopause, as it speeds up the body's own natural healing, balancing

hormones and addressing various systems in the body. Even if you haven't begun to experience any symptoms, Reiki can offer lots of other benefits for your general feeling of well-being, providing an escape from the stresses of everyday life. We are often so busy pleasing everyone else that we tend to forget to take time out for us, but around perimenopause is when we need to reconsider this. It can be very easy to lose who we are as our bodies begin to change and we are trying to cope with hot flushes, mood swings, fatigue, anxiety, pain, low libido, brain fog... Reiki can help with this by helping you find your way back to "you". And, if the mind is calm, the body tends to follow.

# You don't need to change anything about yourself. This is who you are, and it's okay.

UZO ADUBA

# *Get help to stop smoking*

If you smoke, giving up can be easier said than done – especially if menopause symptoms are causing you to feel stressed. But trying to give up really is better for your heart and your oral health – not to mention the risk of cancer and stroke. Smoking can also contribute to the number of hot flushes that we might experience: one seven-year study of 761 women showed that those who gave up nicotine experienced fewer or less intensive hot flushes than those who did not. It's also thought that people who smoke – particularly heavy smokers – might see perimenopause starting earlier than non-smokers. In the early 1960s, another study cited early menopause in 20 per cent of 650 smokers, compared to just 1.7 per cent of 5,000 non-smokers. If you need treatment or advice on how to ditch the cigarettes, then contact your health professional, who can advise on the best course of action.

# Use it or lose it

Keeping our brains and memories functioning well is something we can all benefit from, no matter our age or stage in life. As oestrogen levels decline, this can impact our cognitive ability, and it is thought this may increase our risk of conditions like dementia and Alzheimer's disease. But there are many things we can do to keep the cogs whirring smoothly.

- Who has not heard of Wordle? If you have yet to discover it, head over to www.nytimes.com/games/wordle – and while you're there, there's plenty more word and number-related procrastination material, such as crosswords, sudoku, spelling challenges and other games, to get stuck into.

- Keep learning by taking up a new skill or hobby. Take up painting, drawing or photography; learn a language or musical instrument. This doesn't even have to involve paying an instructor, as there are a multitude of videos and apps to draw upon – ah, the wonders of the twenty-first century!

- Do you remember that game you used to play as a child where you place items on a tray, then cover them with a cloth? Someone removes an item and you must remember what it was. Why not introduce this at home as a rainy Sunday afternoon challenge?

- Free up memory space to retain new information by making use of tech, such as calendar alerts in your phone or sending yourself an email or calling your own voicemail to remind yourself to do something.

- If you normally read fiction, switch genres and choose an autobiography or a non-fiction title about the history of another country. Who knows, you may even discover a new passion or interest along the way.

# Review your treatments

If you do decide to treat your symptoms, whether going down the traditional medical route with HRT, with supplements or via a more holistic treatment method, it's important to review what you're doing and how you're feeling on a regular basis. As perimenopause can last for several years, and your body will continue to change and adjust throughout that time, what is working at one point may not help forever. Keeping a note of your symptoms using a diary (see page 86) will let you see which treatments are making you feel better, for example. And make sure to ask a medical professional to review any treatment or medication every three months to begin with, to discuss any side effects. After that, you may need to be seen less often.

# Find strength in others

If you don't have anyone to talk to about your experiences and symptoms, there may be many others in the same situation as you. You may be quite happy in your own company, and that is of course a perfectly acceptable way of dealing with things! But if you would rather not travel down this road alone, why not think about setting up a community menopause group of your own? It could take the form of a monthly meet-up at a communal hall, in the park or at a local coffee shop. Bring along diet and exercise tips to help each other and details about things you've found useful, and generally offer support and advice to others going through the same thing. You might even start a perimenopause movement!

# Pre-twentieth-century perimenopause

To round off this chapter, let's count ourselves lucky that we're not negotiating our way through perimenopause in different times. Some of the treatments that residents of past time periods endured are quite the eye-opener!

Though the Ancient Greeks were aware of the menopause, back then more than half of women died by age 34, so many simply did not live long enough to experience symptoms.

Fast-forward to the 1800s, when such treatments as electric therapy, opium (a definite no-no, people), the filtered juice of guinea pigs' ovaries, arsenic, thyroid gland extract, vaginal plugs and iced injections were endured. No, thanks!

By the age of the Victorians, women going through "the change" were considered insane; physicians even gave it the term "climacteric insanity". Many doctors believed that removing the ovaries (they no longer worked, after all) would solve all of that. It was also frowned upon for Victorian women to have any kind of sexual desire once they had borne children. By the 1890s women might have been offered a flavoured powder made from cow ovaries. Yummy!

Fortunately for us, the idea that changes in hormone levels were to blame started to be taken seriously by the beginning of the twentieth century. One of the earliest forms of oestrogen replacement was manufactured in the 1940s from the urine of pregnant mares.

While life nowadays is far from perfect, living in the twenty-first century has its benefits. We are very lucky to have medical science on our side and – for most of us – someone who will listen to our concerns and offer us the help that we need.

One day, you will look back and realize all along, you were blooming.

MORGAN HARPER NICHOLS

## Conclusion

So, there you have it. We hope that we have enlightened you about what perimenopause is, when it might appear and how it might present itself. We also hope that you feel reassured of its naturalness and normality. Always remember that you're not alone in this journey, so please don't ever feel embarrassed or awkward about discussing anything with a professional. Your brilliant body will do what it will, but by following the advice and tips given throughout this little book, hopefully it will make it a much smoother ride. Good luck on your journey!

# *Further Reading*

## *Books*

Adams, Kaye and Allen, Vicky, *STILL HOT!: 42 Brilliantly Honest Menopause Stories* (2020, Black & White Publishing)

Chamberlain, Claire, *Self-Kindness: How to Live with Compassion and Create a Life You Love* (2022, Summersdale)

Corinna, Heather, *What Fresh Hell Is This?: Perimenopause, Menopause, Other Indignities, and You* (2021, Hachette Books)

Foxcroft, Louise, *Hot Flushes, Cold Science: The History of the Modern Menopause* (2010, Granta Books)

Green, Wendy, *100 Tips to Help You Through the Menopause: Practical Advice for Every Body* (2022, Summersdale)

Heaton, Michelle, *Hot Flush: Motherhood, the Menopause and Me* (2018, Michael O'Mara)

Hill, Maisie, *Perimenopause Power: Navigating Your Hormones on the Journey* (2021, Bloomsbury)

Kaye, Philippa, *The M Word: Everything You Need to Know About the Menopause* (2022, Summersdale)

McCall, Davina, *Menopausing: The Positive Roadmap to Your Second Spring* (2022, HarperCollins)

Mistry, Mita, *How to Understand and Deal with Social Anxiety: Everything You Need to Know to Manage Social Anxiety* (2022, Summersdale)

Mosconi, Lisa, *The XX Brain: The Groundbreaking Science Empowering Women to Maximize Cognitive Health and Prevent Alzheimer's Disease* (2020, Penguin)

Newson, Louise, *Preparing for the Perimenopause and Menopause* (2021, Penguin UK)

O'Brien, Dominic, *You Can Have an Amazing Memory: Learn Life-Changing Techniques and Tips from the Memory Maestro* (2016, Watkins Media)

## Magazines
*Menopause Matters: www.menopausematters.co.uk*

## Bra Fitting Advice
*www.freyalingerie.com*

*www.booborbust.com*

*Bra Size Calculator (with conversions for the US, Europe, Australia and NZ): www.calculator.net/bra-size-calculator.html*

## Websites
*The Migraine Trust: www.migrainetrust.org*

Counselling Directory: www.counselling-directory.org.uk (UK only)

The Menopause Charity, Menopause Facts, Advice and Support: www.themenopausecharity.org

Menopause and Me: www.menopauseandme.co.uk – also contains a handy checklist to use to talk to a medical professional

Website of menopause expert Dr Louise Newson: www.newsonhealth.co.uk

British Menopause Society: www.thebms.org.uk

Menopause Cafe: www.menopausecafe.net

Website of BIWOC advocate Katara McCarty: www.kataramccarty.com (with a link to the Exhale app for Black, Indigenous and Women of Colour)

Queer Menopause: www.queermenopause.com

Help and support from the NHS: www.nhs.uk/conditions/menopause/help-and-support/

## Podcasts and apps
BBC Woman's Hour on BBC Sounds: www.bbc.co.uk/sounds

www.blackgirlsguidetosurvivingmenopause.com

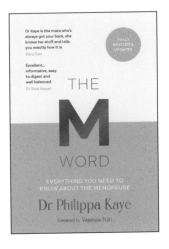

**THE M WORD**
*Everything You Need to Know About the Menopause*

**Dr Philippa Kaye**

Paperback

ISBN:
978-1-80007-831-4

The menopause does not have to mean the end of your libido, of sex, of work, or of feeling like who you used to be.

*The M Word* is a complete one-stop guide to the perimenopause and menopause, covering everything from understanding symptoms and managing relationships to figuring out which treatments really work.

Have you enjoyed this book? If so, find us on Facebook at **Summersdale Publishers**, on Twitter at **@Summersdale** and on Instagram at **@summersdalebooks** and get in touch. We'd love to hear from you!

## www.summersdale.com